Diabetic retinopathy

A guide for diabetes care teams

William D. Alexander FRCP

Consultant Physician (Diabetes)
Western General Hospital NHS Trust
Edinburgh

**Blackwell
Science**

© 1998 by
Blackwell Science Ltd
Editorial Offices:
Osney Mead, Oxford OX2 0EL
25 John Street, London WC1N 2BL
23 Ainslie Place, Edinburgh EH3 6AJ
350 Main Street, Malden
  MA 02148 5018, USA
54 University Street, Carlton
  Victoria 3053, Australia
10, rue Casimir Delavigne
  75006 Paris, France

Other Editorial Offices:
Blackwell Wissenschafts-Verlag GmbH
Kurfürstendamm 57
10707 Berlin, Germany

Blackwell Science KK
MG Kodenmacho Building
7–10 Kodenmacho Nihombashi
Chuo-ku, Tokyo 104, Japan

The right of the Author to be
identified as the Author of this Work
has been asserted in accordance
with the Copyright, Designs and
Patents Act 1988.

First published 1998

Set by Excel Typesetters Co., Hong Kong
Printed and bound in Great Britain
at the University Press, Cambridge

The Blackwell Science logo is a
trade mark of Blackwell Science Ltd,
registered at the United Kingdom
Trade Marks Registry

DISTRIBUTORS

Marston Book Services Ltd
PO Box 269
Abingdon, Oxon OX14 4YN
(Orders: Tel: 01235 465500
        Fax: 01235 465555)

USA
Blackwell Science, Inc.
Commerce Place
350 Main Street
Malden, MA 02148 5018
(Orders: Tel: 800 759 6102
        781 388 8250
        Fax: 781 388 8255)

Canada
Login Brothers Book Company
324 Saulteaux Crescent
Winnipeg, Manitoba R3J 3T2
(Orders: Tel: 204 837-2987

Australia
Blackwell Science Pty Ltd
54 University Street
Carlton, Victoria 3053
(Orders: Tel: 3 9347 0300
        Fax: 3 9347 5001)

A catalogue record for this title
is available from the British Library and the
Library of Congress

ISBN 0-632-05171-X

For further information on
Blackwell Science, visit our website:
www.blackwell-science.com

Contents

Contents

Preface

Diabetes care is an increasingly multidisciplinary specialty involving many professionals in varied sectors of health-care structures. All those involved in diabetes care will encounter patients who are concerned about retinopathy and many people who have been affected by the condition. This book is *not* intended to be a comprehensive review of retinopathy but to provide an outline of the disease, its importance, the screening process and the criteria for referral for treatment that can prevent progression to visual loss. I hope that at least some sections will be of interest to all involved health-care professionals, from students and specialty trainees to experienced practitioners in general medicine, diabetes, ophthalmology and optometry, both in the hospital and primary care settings. I hope that it will be helpful to them in understanding and managing people threatened, or coping, with this important condition.

The illustrations, including the common nondiabetic ophthalmic conditions, are based upon the experience of a provincial diabetes care unit and I would like particularly to acknowledge, and express my gratitude for, the support of Bill David of the retinal photographic department of Queen Mary's Hospital, Sidcup, Kent. I would also like to thank the Department of Medical Photography at the Western General Hospital, Edinburgh, and Mr Ken Swa, Ophthalmologist, at the Edinburgh Eye Pavilion for their support in providing some of the photographs.

Introduction and aims

Diabetes mellitus is a common condition with an increasing incidence and prevalence. There is no such thing as 'mild diabetes' or 'just a bit of sugar'; all types carry a high morbidity and mortality both of which can be significantly influenced by good medical care. It is therefore of great importance that all medical practitioners, and other health-care professionals, are aware of the needs and expectations of people with diabetes and the expected standards of modern methods of diagnosis and management of the condition and its complications.

Diabetic retinopathy is one of the most feared of the microvascular complications because it may lead to blindness if not detected and adequately treated sufficiently early. Failure to detect it at an early and treatable stage may lead to loss of vision, and such neglect may now be considered an indefensible case for litigation.

Efficient and effective screening for diabetic retinopathy is an essential part of any diabetic annual review. It requires considerable skill and experience. Such skills not only relate to the detection and management of diabetic eye disease, but also to the management of the diabetes as a whole. This will include the management of the metabolic state, the detection and management of other associated microvascular complications, and other general risk factors for vascular disease. All these factors are relevant for successful management of diabetic eye disease and prevention of blindness.

This book is designed to help update practitioners in this important aspect of diabetes care. It is not designed to make everyone self-sufficient in the screening and management of this complicated subject, but to provide them with information and insight to ensure that the necessary processes and expertise are made available to everyone with diabetes by the appropriate available specialists. Without specific training primary care physicians generally are unlikely to be able to reliably screen for retinopathy because of lack of equipment, expertise and exposure. They are essential however to ensure that their patients avail themselves of local screening programmes and are important in dealing with the other relevant nonophthalmological factors which include the various other medical and psychosocial implications of the development of retinopathy to the persons developing the condition.

Most localities now have multidisciplinary specialty diabetes care teams, yet not all people with diabetes are availing themselves of formal review and care to the standards expected. Primary care remains an essential element in trying to correct this deficiency. They need not necessarily do it themselves but should be able to ensure that it is done. Treatment for diabetic eye disease, if detected early, is now successful and together we should be able to significantly reduce the threat of blindness to our diabetic patients.

1 Diabetic retinopathy: epidemiology and classification

Diabetic retinopathy continues to threaten blindness for people with diabetes and is the commonest cause of visual loss registration amongst people of working age. It is hoped that such statistics will soon be seen to have been improved by better screening, earlier recognition and timely treatment. Everyone with diabetes is at risk, however 'mild' the metabolic disorder may be perceived to be, and it is therefore essential that all members of diabetes care teams are aware of the importance of this microvascular complication. All professionals involved in diabetic eye screening should be skilled in the ability to detect and recognize retinopathies of differing severity and this chapter outlines some of the epidemiology of the condition and also its classification.

Epidemiology, pathophysiology, and natural history

The occurrence and severity of diabetic retinopathy is related to the duration of diabetes and to the degree of metabolic control. It is unusual to find signs of retinopathy in type 1 insulin-dependent diabetes mellitus (IDDM) within the first 5 years and rarely severe within 10 years, but then its incidence increases rapidly. Whereas retinopathy may be present in only 2% after 2 years, after 20 years this figure is greater than 90% and 50% of these may be of the severe proliferative type (Fig. 1.1). In type 2 noninsulin-dependent diabetes mellitus (NIDDM) the situation is different because NIDDM may be present but undiagnosed for many years. As many as 20% may have signs of retinopathy at the time of diagnosis and this may be severe and sight threatening. Retinal examination is therefore an essential part of the examination of any person with newly diagnosed NIDDM.

In broad terms diabetic retinopathy is the result of an ischaemic process involving the microvasculature of the retina.

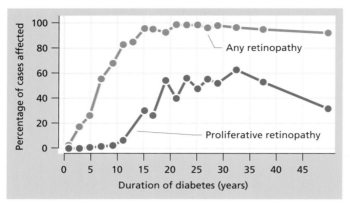

Figure 1.1 Frequency of retinopathies by duration of diabetes in insulin-dependent diabetes mellitus diagnosed before the age of 30 years.

Although the exact process is not fully understood, persistent hyperglycaemia is the likely cause and sets off a chain of events in the retina that are both anatomical and biochemical. These changes lead to capillary occlusion and, depending upon the degree of severity, to ischaemia, capillary leakage and attempts by the retina to correct the situation by new vessel formation (Fig. 1.2). The stages of diabetic retinopathy are shown in Fig. 1.3.

The first signs of retinopathy are the development of micro-aneurysms and small haemorrhages, seen as red dots and blots, which occur at the site of capillary occlusion, dilatation and rupture (Fig. 1.4). The numbers will vary and they may come and go depending upon the extent of the areas of ischaemia and the degree of control of precipitating factors. Further abnormalities lead to increased permeability of the capillary walls through which there is leakage of lipids producing 'hard' exudates, seen as yellowish streaks, rings or blots (Fig. 1.5). If such exudates occur near the macula (maculopathy), or within the temporal vascular arcade and therefore threaten to affect the macula, they may require laser treatment to prevent significant and irreversible visual loss. This is the type of change that most commonly leads to visual loss in the person with Type 2 diabetes (NIDDM). For laser treatment to be most effective it is important that such changes

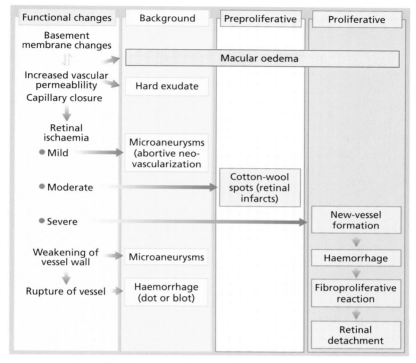

Figure 1.2 Scheme of pathological changes of diabetic retinopathy.

are detected before there has been any effect on vision and in this respect screening is essential.

More extensive ischaemia leads to increasing numbers of the above changes and also to the appearance of retinal infarcts seen as 'cotton wool spots' or 'soft' exudates (Fig. 1.6). In response to increasing ischaemia, venous changes, seen as beading and looping occur. Retinal attempts at angioneogenesis then lead to intraretinal microvascular abnormalities (IRMAs) (see Fig. 1.10). This process may further lead to proliferative new vessel formation either on the disc (NVD) or elsewhere on the retina (NVE). This proliferative type of retinopathy is most commonly seen in longstanding Type 1 diabetes (IDDM). Such vessels are fragile

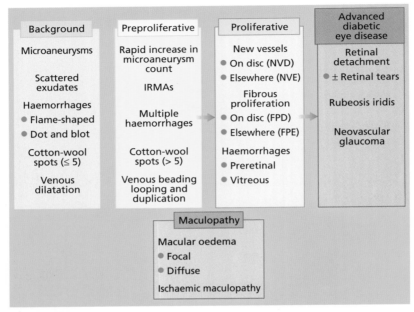

Background	Preproliferative	Proliferative	Advanced diabetic eye disease
Microaneurysms	Rapid increase in microaneurysm count	New vessels ● On disc (NVD) ● Elsewhere (NVE)	Retinal detachment ● ± Retinal tears
Scattered exudates	IRMAs	Fibrous proliferation	Rubeosis iridis
Haemorrhages ● Flame-shaped ● Dot and blot	Multiple haemorrhages	● On disc (FPD) ● Elsewhere (FPE)	Neovascular glaucoma
Cotton-wool spots (≤ 5)	Cotton-wool spots (> 5)	Haemorrhages ● Preretinal	
Venous dilatation	Venous beading looping and duplication	● Vitreous	

Maculopathy

Macular oedema
● Focal
● Diffuse

Ischaemic maculopathy

Figure 1.3 Stages of diabetic retinopathy.

Figure 1.4 Microaneurysms (close up).

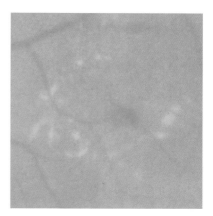

Figure 1.5 Exudates (close up).

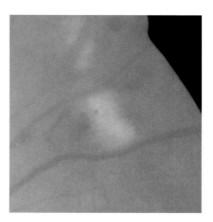

Figure 1.6 Cotton wool spot (close up).

and grow out from the retina and if not treated will bleed causing a preretinal or vitreous haemorrhage. If still not treated such a haemorrhage, which leads to loss of vision, will subsequently develop into fibrous scarring, which as it contracts will detach the retina. Further new vessel proliferation, as well as repeating this process, may spread anteriorly and affect the iris (rubeosis iridis) and this subsequently can produce painful rubeotic glaucoma that may require enucleation of the eye.

Types of diabetic retinopathy

Diabetic retinopathy may be classified into nonproliferative, proliferative and advanced retinopathies. Nonproliferative retinopathies include background retinopathy, the sight threatening maculopathies and preproliferative retinopathy. The risk of nonproliferative retinopathy progressing to proliferative change depends upon the extent of the underlying ischaemic process. New vessels on the optic disc (NVD) or elsewhere on the retina (NVE) characterize proliferative retinopathy. If proliferative retinopathy is left untreated it will develop into advanced eye disease and blindness.

Non-proliferative retinopathy

Background retinopathy (Fig. 1.7)
Background retinopathy is the term used for the early changes of diabetic retinopathy and includes the following features:
- Microaneurysms: retinal capillary microaneurysms appear as red dots.
- Haemorrhages: appear as blots or flame shaped streaks. In background retinopathy they are small and few in number.
- Exudates: yellow, well defined areas that appear as blots, rings, or streaks depending upon the site of the capillary leakage. The retinopathy should be classified as 'background with maculopathy' if they occur near or in the macula.

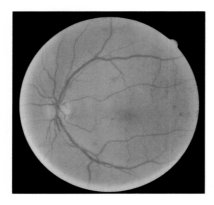

Figure 1.7 Mild background diabetic retinopathy.

- Cotton wool spots: small, fluffy, white, roundish areas that represent accumulation of axoplasm at the margin of infarction. They are few in number in background retinopathy but more numerous (>5) when a feature of preproliferative change.

Maculopathy (Fig. 1.8)

Maculopathy accounts for the majority of cases of blindness in diabetes because it is the predominant cause in cases of the numerically more common type 2 diabetes, NIDDM. Visual deterioration due to maculopathy may be the presenting symptom in longstanding undiagnosed NIDDM and treatment at such a late stage may then be difficult or ineffective.

- Exudative maculopathy (Fig. 1.8). Circinate exudates (as in background retinopathy) may be seen in the temporal vessel arcades or at the edge of the macula. Nearer the fovea they may appear as streaks or spokes. They are due to focal capillary leakage. This type of maculopathy responds to laser treatment.
- Macular oedema. Diffuse vascular leakage causes macula oedema. It is difficult to detect with direct ophthalmoscopy but is suggested if there is a marked, uncorrectable reduction in visual acuity without opacity of the media.
- Ischaemic maculopathy. This is suggested if there are clusters of microaneurysms and haemorrhages with other signs of central retinal ischaemia (white vessels and an empty avascular appearance) with reduced visual acuity.

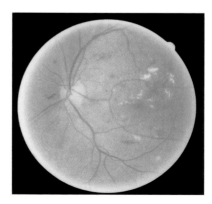

Figure 1.8 Background retinopathy with circinate exudates and maculopathy.

Preproliferative retinopathy (Figs 1.9 & 1.10)

Preproliferative changes occur as capillary closure becomes more widespread and, as well as the signs of extensive background retinopathy, include the features listed below.

- Multiple cotton wool spots (>5).
- Larger blotchy haemorrhages.
- IRMAs. These appear as small areas of very fine abnormal blood vessels lying flat within the retina, unlike the new vessels of proliferative retinopathy that appear to grow out from the veins.
- Venous abnormalities. Beading of the veins may appear like a string of sausages; venous loops or reduplication may also occur.

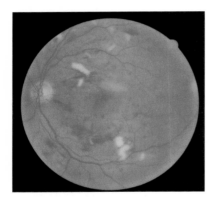

Figure 1.9 Preproliferative retinopathy in a man with diabetes and hypertension. Background retinopathy changes plus multiple cotton wool spots, haemorrhages and venous change.

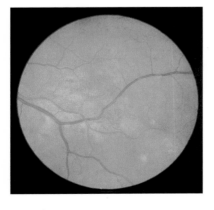

Figure 1.10 Intraretinal microvascular abnormalities.

Proliferative retinopathy (Figs 1.11–1.14)

In response to increasing retinal nonperfusion, neovascularization may occur with new blood vessels growing out from the retinal vascular arcades and extending onto the vitreous. They are extremely fragile and if untreated cause preretinal or vitreous haemorrhage and thereby lead to loss of vision. This type of sight

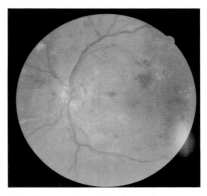

Figure 1.11 Proliferative retinopathy. New vessels on the disc and a background of haemorrhages, exudates, cotton wool spots and preproliferative changes with venous angiopathy and intraretinal microvascular abnormalities. Empty, ghost vessels denote further retinal ischaemia. This is a 40-year-old man, newly diagnosed as having noninsulin-dependent diabetes mellitus (NIDDM) when admitted for routine hernia surgery. *It is essential to screen all newly diagnosed patients with NIDDM.*

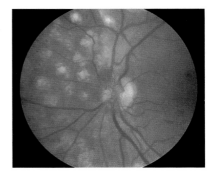

Figure 1.12 Proliferative retinopathy. New vessels arising from the optic disc and peripheral scars from laser photocoagulation treatment.

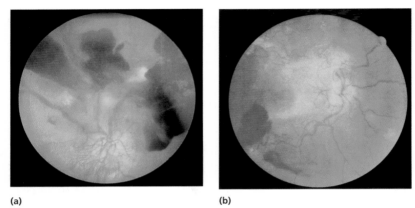

(a)   (b)

Figure 1.13 Proliferative retinopathy with preretinal haemorrhage from bleeding new vessels.

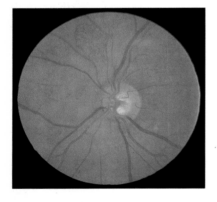

Figure 1.14 New vessel formation elsewhere (NVE), e.g. in areas other than the optic disc.

threatening retinopathy is the one most likely to occur in long-standing IDDM.

• NVD: new vessels arising from vessels on the optic disc, or
• NVE: from vessels elsewhere on the retina.

Proliferative retinopathy requires urgent laser treatment to prevent bleeding and irretrievable loss of vision.

Advanced diabetic retinopathy (Figs 1.15 & 1.16)

Proliferative retinopathy, if left untreated, produces a sequence

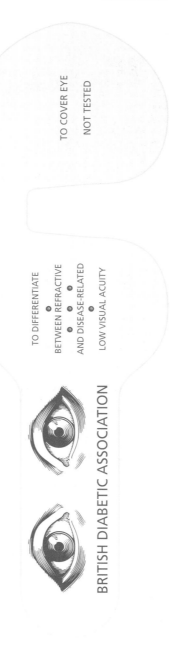

TO COVER EYE
NOT TESTED

TO DIFFERENTIATE
BETWEEN REFRACTIVE
AND DISEASE-RELATED
LOW VISUAL ACUITY

BRITISH DIABETIC ASSOCIATION

Figure 2.2 Pinhole aid for testing corrected visual acuity.

Snellen chart (Fig. 2.3)

This consists of a series of letters in rows of different sizes. Each row has a designated number. The row numbers, from top to bottom, are usually 60, 36, 24, 18, 12, 9, 6. These numbers represent the distance (in metres) at which someone with normal vision should be able to read that line. The visual acuity is expressed as a ratio of the test distance (6 m or 20 feet) over the number of the smallest line that can be read. Standard normal vision is 6/6 (or 20/20 if expressed in feet). If a person cannot read the top line (i.e. their vision is worse than 6/60) they can

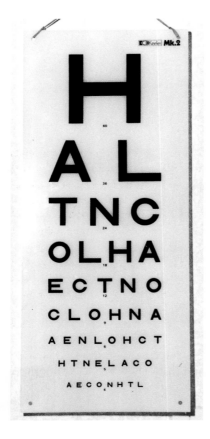

Figure 2.3 Snellen chart for measuring visual acuity.

move nearer the chart. If readable at 3 m acuity would be 3/60, or at 1 m, 1/60. With normal visual fields, vision of 6/60 or worse in both eyes warrants registration as partially sighted and <3/60 as blind (if the visual fields are restricted, people can be registered at better levels of acuity).

If the acuity is worse than 1/60 the person may be asked to count fingers, and, if unable to do so, to detect hand movement. Worse than this may require testing to see whether a light source can be detected or whether there is not even any perception of light.

Recording visual acuity	
Standard visual acuity	6/6
Partial sight registration	<6/60
Blind registration	<3/60
Counting fingers	CF
Hand movements	HM
Perception of light	PL
No light perception	NPL

Pupil dilation (mydriasis)

It is essential to dilate the pupils prior to ophthalmoscopy. Older people and those with longstanding diabetes often have smallish pupils. Diabetic retinopathy and potentially sight-threatening changes may only be present temporal to the macula, an area that is impossible to see through small undilated pupils. A reliable view of the retina cannot therefore be obtained without mydriasis.

Tropicamide 0.5 or 1% eye drops (Fig. 2.4) should be instilled into each eye. The risk of precipitating acute glaucoma is remote but patients should be asked if there is any history of the same. Ophthalmological advice regarding safety should be sought if there is such a history and/or if there have been certain types of previous intraocular surgery.

Tropicamide pupil dilation will cause blurring of vision, which will last for several hours. Patients should be warned of this and be instructed to avoid driving at such a time.

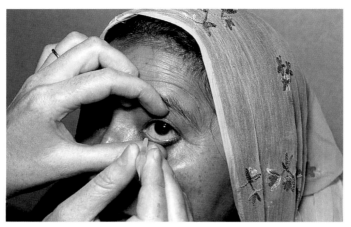

(a)

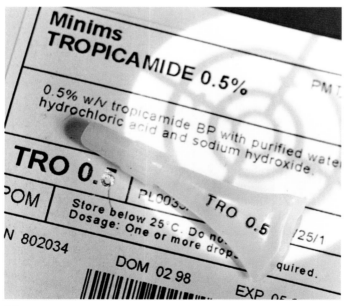

(b)

Figure 2.4 (a) Dilating the pupil of the eye with mydriatic eye drops.
(b) Tropicamide eye drops.

Ophthalmoscopy

The ophthalmoscope

Slit lamp biomicroscopy is the ideal method for examining the retina. This is not available to most diabetes care teams and it is the monocular direct ophthalmoscope that is usually used (Fig. 2.5). It is not easy and requires considerable skill, training and practice.

Ophthalmoscope light sources may have a variable number of different lenses depending upon the degree of sophistication

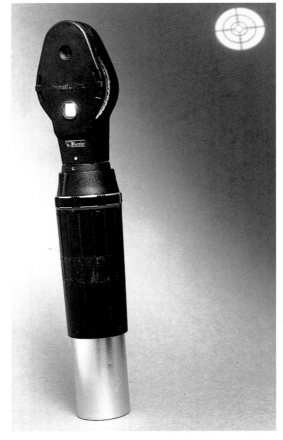

Figure 2.5 (a) A direct ophthalmoscope.

(a)

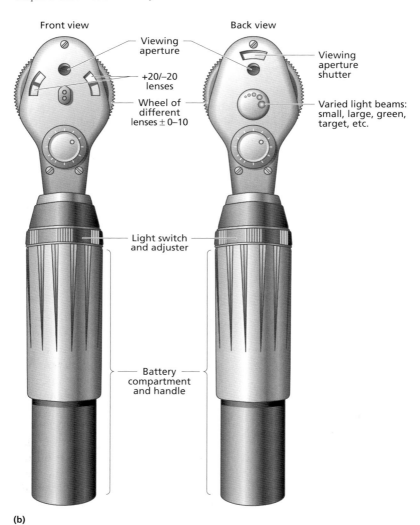

(b)

Figure 2.5 *Continued.* (b) Details of the components of a direct ophthalmoscope.

(and cost) of the instrument used. All will shine a white light, the
intensity of which can be adjusted. Some will have a series of
lenses that can alter the size of arc of light. There may also be a
green filter, which is useful to enhance the appearance and clarity
of blood vessels and microaneurysms.

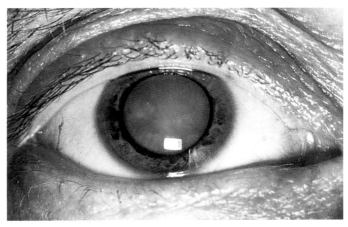

Figure 2.6 Cataract.

All ophthalmoscopes have a rack of lenses on a wheel, which can be adjusted to obtain a clear view depending upon the refractive errors of the eyes of the examiner and the patient. These numbers may be black (+ lenses) or red (– lenses). The examiner may find it easier to wear his/her own glasses while using the instrument. If patients have extreme refractive errors they can be asked to keep their glasses on, this is useful when examining the optic disc but often produces excessive reflection when examining the rest of the retina.

Ophthalmoscopy should be done in a darkened room.

Patients should be asked to focus on a distant object. To enable such fixation the examiner should hold the ophthalmoscope in the right hand and use the right eye to examine the patient's right eye and vice versa for the left. The free hand may need to be laid gently on the patient's forehead with the thumb on the eyebrow and eye lid to prevent interference from eyelashes and keep the eyelid retracted. The opthalmoscope is best held with the hand wrapped around its 'body' and the tip of the index finger on the adjustable wheel of lenses.

The ophthalmoscope lens rack should be set on '0' and held at least one foot away with the light shining on the patient's pupil. A red reflection (reflex) should be observed from the retina. If absent, it suggests there is a corneal opacity or cataract (Fig. 2.6) in the way. Initially holding the ophthalmoscope at a distance from the eye enables the examiner to gradually move nearer, while looking through the instrument, and thereby, initially, to focus on the cornea and lens and to detect abnormalities such as cataract.

Moving closer the retina becomes visible; the ophthalmoscope should be focused by moving the rack of lenses until a clear image is seen.

Examining the retina (Fig. 2.7)

The optic disc is a good point of reference at which to start. It is the channel through which the retinal nerve fibres leave the eye via the optic nerve. The central retinal artery and vein also enter and leave at this point. The retinal arteries and veins spread out over the superior and inferior temporal and the superior and inferior nasal retinal quadrants. The retinal capillary bed, where diabetic retinopathy starts, extends throughout the retina except at the fovea, which lies at the very centre of the macula.

The macula is the central area of the retina and lies temporal to the optic disc between the main superior and inferior temporal vascular arcades. It looks redder than the surrounding retina.

Examination of the retina with the ophthalmoscope should begin at the optic disc. New blood vessels of proliferative retino-pathy may occur here (NVD). They can be distinguished from normal blood vessels because they are thin and grow forward

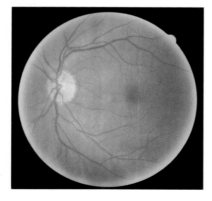

Figure 2.7 Normal optic fundus.

rather than following the normal flat course of other vessels on the retina. They may appear as tufts or arcades. The ophthalmo-scope may need to be moved slightly away from the eye to bring NVD into clearer focus.

The retinal vessels and each quadrant of the retina should then be carefully inspected for changes of diabetic retinopathy and finally the macula and fovea examined carefully for changes of diabetic maculopathy or age-related degenerative change.

The quadrants can be examined either by the examiner manoeuvring the ophthalmoscope light around the retina with the patient's gaze remaining on a fixed object or alternatively by asking the patient to look serially up, down, right and left while the examiners gaze remains fixed. For the macula to be seen the patient can be asked to look directly into the light of the ophthalmoscope.

Findings should be carefully checked and documented. Decisions regarding the necessity for referral should be made. The management and implications should be explained and discussed with the patient. A date for the next examination should be arranged.

Difficulties with ophthalmoscopy
Inadequately charged batteries
Room not darkened
Pupil inadequately dilated
'High myopic' patient (examine with patient wearing his or her glasses)
Cataract
Inexperienced examiner

3 Screening for diabetic retinopathy

Standards

The following factors may be considered as essentials for diabetic eye screening (British Diabetic Association 1997).

- Screening programmes sensitive to local circumstances should be available to all people with diabetes on an annual basis whether they are cared for in hospitals or in the community.
- Screening achieves worthwhile health gains provided that the sensitivity is high enough and patient compliance is good. The screening programme must monitor both sensitivity and specificity in order to ensure adequate performance in practice and yet protect ophthalmology departments from unnecessary referrals.
- Significant training implications should be recognized and facilities and resources made available.
- For any screening programme to be effective, an efficient call and recall system is essential.
- More than one method of screening may be required to serve the population most effectively.
- Annual screening intervals are recommended.
- Efficiency and effectiveness of the screening should be audited.

The generally accepted gold standard for screening for diabetic retinopathy would be for all patients with diabetes to be seen annually by an ophthalmologist with a special interest in the condition using the equipment necessary for reliable fundoscopy (slit-lamp biomicroscopy, direct and indirect ophthalmoscopy and retinal photography). This however, is not logistically possible in the UK. Furthermore it is important not to swamp ophthalmology departments with screening commitments as this may diminish their ability to offer timely treatment and therefore be counterproductive.

Specialist diabetes centres and specialist diabetologists will usually have sufficient training, experience and available equipment to screen reliably, but will not see everyone with diabetes in the locality. Often they will see less than 50%. The other 50% will be seen by either their primary care physician or nobody at all.

Primary care physicians, who are, at least in theory, able to identify all people with diabetes, do not usually have the training, experience, or the equipment to screen reliably and may miss up to 65% of significant retinopathies.

Therefore, if a significant impact is to be made on the incidence of blindness due to diabetic retinopathy, an agreed formal diabetic retinopathy screening programme, using one or more of the methods of proven efficacy, is necessary in all localities. This need is recognized by the Department of Health and the BDA.

The UK Department of Health and British Diabetic Association St Vincent Taskforce for Diabetes final report
Preventing blindness in diabetes (visual impairment subgroup)
Key facts:
- Diabetic retinopathy is the most common cause of blindness in the population of working age in the UK
- The risk of retinopathy in people with insulin dependent diabetes mellitus is halved by intensified diabetic control
- Regular (annual) screening for retinopathy detects those at risk before visual symptoms occur and when treatment outcome is optimal
- Treatment can prevent blindness in 90% of those at risk if applied early and adequately

Priority needs:
- A formally structured retinopathy screening programme for all patients in all localities, using one or more of the methods of proven efficacy
- Access to specialist diagnostic, treatment and counselling services for those screening positive
- Local registration, documentation and care plans for regular patient review
- Adequate provision of support, education and retraining for the visually handicapped

---

What are 'methods of proven efficacy'?

Most localities in the UK now have, or are developing, a formal diabetic retinopathy screening programme which involves a combination of specialist diabetes physicians, specifically trained and accredited optometrists and ophthalmic medical practitioners (OMPs) performing dilated ophthalmoscopy, and the use of retinal cameras. Such schemes are set up with the agreement of local specialist ophthalmologists with whom referral guidelines for further assessment and treatment have to be agreed.

Dilated ophthalmoscopy (Fig. 3.1)

Dilation of the pupil is essential for ophthalmoscopy. Retinal examination is best carried out using slit lamp biomicroscopy but may be performed by indirect or direct ophthalmoscopy. Direct ophthalmoscopy is the method most commonly used but is only as reliable as the person performing the examination. It is essential that anyone with the responsibility for ophthalmoscopic (and camera) diabetic eye screening is adequately trained.

Formal screening programmes may involve optometrists. Optometrists are conveniently situated in the community and therefore easily accessible. They have specific training in the examination of the eye and examine fundi day in and day out. Provided that they have further initial and ongoing training specifically regarding diabetic eye disease they are reliable for diabetic retinopathy screening.

Training to screen for diabetic retinopathy should include the following

1 The structure of the local diabetes care services

2 General medical aspects of diabetes:
   • pathology and epidemiology
   • treatment and monitoring
   • importance of patient education
   • nonophthalmic complications of diabetes
   • other medical problems that may coexist

3 Ophthalmic aspects of diabetes:
   • changes in refraction (myopic and hypermetropic shifts)
   • iris and rubeosis
   • cataract
   • classification of diabetic retinopathy and risk factors
   • recognition and grading of various forms of retinopathy and their risks to vision
   • referral criteria and treatments for retinopathy
   • the use and complications of mydriatics

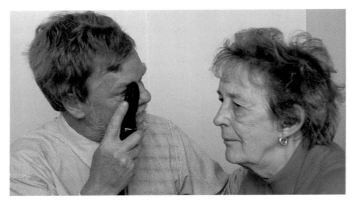

Figure 3.1 Direct ophthalmoscopy.

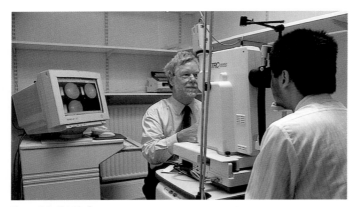

Figure 3.2 Retinal camera.

Retinal photography (Fig. 3.2)

The use of retinal cameras has been proven to be cost effective and to have a high sensitivity and specificity. The recent introduction of digital imaging cameras has been a further advance. Retinal photography can be used as a back up to ophthalmoscopy or as the primary means of screening. Ideally both methods should be used. Training and accreditation for screeners using cameras is as essential as it is for ophthalmoscopy. The camera screening unit can either be static and on one site or housed in a van and be mobile around the locality. Dilation of the pupil is essential. Although multiple stereoscopic views to cover the whole retina are the ideal, this is not practical for routine screening and a single picture to include the disc, major temporal vascular arcades and macula is usually taken. This covers the area most commonly affected by potentially sight threatening retinopathy. Either 35 mm or Polaroid film may be used unless a digital imaging camera is available.

Retinal films need to be seen and reported by ophthalmologists, or alternatively by the diabetologist who can then discuss positive findings directly with the ophthalmologists, thereby potentially decreasing patient and health service costs and time expenditure in borderline cases. Photographs are also very useful educationally, both to patients and professionals.

Essential roles of primary care in ensuring patients attend for eye screening

It is important that all people with diabetes are aware of the importance of eye screening and know why and how to access the screening process. The following may be helpful in ensuring this occurs.

> When a patient with diabetes is seen:
> - Ensure they are aware of the seriousness of diabetic eye disease and of the need for regular eye examination regardless of the absence of any symptoms
> - Make sure they are aware of the local eye screening programme and how to access it
> - Explain that such eye screening examinations are paid for by the NHS and there will be no charge to them
> - Give them a leaflet explaining the scheme (see example, p. 32)
> - Ensure that they attend

Awareness posters and educational leaflets in surgeries are also useful and are available from the BDA (Fig. 3.3).

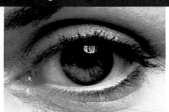

Eye problems caused by diabetes can usually be prevented by simple treatment.

People with diabetes need to have their eyes examined and tested regularly.

Ask your doctor to arrange for the back of your eyes to be examined every year and if you are diabetic free eye tests are available from your local optician.

For advice and details of all the information available from the BDA, write to:-

BRITISH DIABETIC ASSOCIATION
10 Queen Anne Street, London W1M OBD. Tel: 071-323 1531

LIFTING THE SHADOW OF DIABETES

Figure 3.3 British Diabetic Association poster.

Organization of diabetic eye screening in primary care

Many patients with diabetes will be seen only in primary care or may not be formally recorded at all as having diabetes on a practice register. The latter are at particular risk of falling through the screening net.

The following suggestions may be useful

1 Maintain a practice register of all people with diabetes. Check that the numbers match the expected prevalence for the locality.

2 When a diabetic patient is seen for review:
- Ensure that he or she is aware of the importance of diabetic eye disease and of the need for regular eye examination even though there may not be any symptoms.
- Check that such an examination has been performed within the last 12 months.
- Make sure patients are aware of the local eye screening programme (if available) and how to access it. Give him or her a leaflet explaining the scheme (see example below).
- If eye examination *has not* been performed, arrange such an examination as soon as possible either with the local formal screening programme or, if not available, perform such an examination (if trained) and/or refer to the local specialist diabetes service.
- If eye examination *has* been performed, check result and that appropriate action has been taken.
- Confirm and/or arrange date for next eye screening.

3 When eye screening result is known
If normal:
Record result and arrange or confirm next eye screening date.
If abnormal:
Explain findings and implications to patient.
Ensure appropriately referred to ophthalmology *if indicated.*
Ensure general assessment of diabetes control and associated vascular risk factors and treat further as necessary.
Refer to specialist diabetic clinic as per local arrangements.
Arrange next screening date as indicated.

4 Audit. Recording screening visits and referrals on audit files for annual analysis is an important way of ensuring that the process of efficient and effective eye screening is occurring and correcting any deficiencies.

Awareness posters in surgeries are also useful and are available from the BDA (Fig. 3.3).

Sample letter for patients attending eye screening programmes*

I am writing to be sure that you are aware of the local diabetic eye screening service. We want to be sure that you know about this and that you make certain you attend every year. This has been developed especially for people with diabetes, it is paid for by the NHS and there will be no charge to yourself—it is free.

Remember that diabetes can cause eye problems. If these are not found early enough (this can be before you notice any change in eyesight) and treated, they can lead to blindness. It is therefore very important that you have this special eye examination each year so that we can pick up any problems that may be there and arrange treatment to stop them getting worse.

The eye test will include a test of your eyesight. Drops will then be put into the eyes to enable an examination of the back of the eye (the retina), to check for any diabetic changes. Results will be sent to your doctor/diabetes clinic and referral for treatment made if necessary.

Some people find it difficult to drive after the eye drops and examination, as they can cause blurred vision for up to 4 h. You should therefore try and make arrangements not to drive yourself to and from this test.

Everyone with diabetes should be sure to make an arrangement to have this special eye examination done once a year. It will only *not* be necessary for you do so if you are already attending the hospital's specialist eye clinic.

This is a most important service especially for you. Please make sure you use it and help beat diabetic eye disease!

* Such a letter will need adapting according to the local scheme. For example, if optometry based, it should include a list of participating optometrists.

Summary

All primary care physicians should ensure that:

- They have a register of all patients in their practice who have diabetes.
- Every patient is aware, and included in, the local eye screening programme.
- That each and everyone has, annually, a formal eye examination using a method(s) of proven efficacy (specifically trained ophthalmoscopist and/or retinal photography).
- The result of the screening is seen, discussed with the patient and appropriate, timely referral is made to an ophthalmologist if indicated.
- Other risk factors are identified and dealt with and/or referred to the specialist diabetes team as indicated.

4   Referral criteria

People screening positive, i.e. those found to have diabetic retinopathy, will all require some further specialist assessment. In some instances (see below) this will require referral to an ophthalmology department for specific treatment of the eye disease. Whether or not this is the case, all people will require explanation of the findings and discussion about the metabolic control of the diabetes itself and consideration of other risk factors, complications and treatments of a general nature.

Below are outlined the generally agreed criteria and timings for referral to specialist ophthalmologists for specific treatment to the eye*.

Sight-threatening lesions requiring *immediate* referral for urgent attention

1 Proliferative retinopathy:
- new vessels at the optic disc (NVD)
- new vessels elsewhere on the retina (NVE)
- preretinal haemorrhages
- fibrous tissue

2 Advanced diabetic eye disease:
- vitreous haemorrhage and/or
- fibrous tissue and/or
- recent retinal detachment and/or
- new vessels on the iris (rubeosis iridis)

Potentially sight-threatening lesions requiring early referral for attention as soon as possible

1 Preproliferative retinopathy:
- venous abnormalities (beading, loops, reduplication) and/or
- multiple haemorrhages and/or

* Based upon the recommendations of the Retinopathy Working Party. A protocol for screening for diabetic retinopathy in Europe.

- multiple cotton wool spots and/or
- intraretinal microvascular abnormalities (IRMAs)

2 Nonproliferative retinopathy with macular involvement:
- haemorrhages and/or exudates within one disc diameter of the macula with or without reduced vision
- reduced visual acuity not corrected by pinhole or glasses (suggests macular oedema)

3 Nonproliferative retinopathy without macular involvement:
- large circinate or plaque exudate(s) within the major temporal vascular arcades

4 Any other abnormality that cannot be interpreted with reasonable certainty

Non-sight threatening lesions that do *not* require referral to ophthalmology but can safely be rescreened in 6–12 months
- Cotton wool spots in small numbers not associated with preproliferative features
- Occasional haemorrhages and/or microaneurysms (red dots and blots) and/or exudates not within one disc diameter of the macular area (Drusen may sometimes be confused with exudates. Drusen, if not associated with other signs of age-related macular degeneration, are not considered important)

Proliferative retinopathy should be considered an emergency, requires immediate attention and therefore an urgent telephone call for personal discussion with the ophthalmologist.

Many specialist diabetologists will offer an intermediary screening service for primary care practitioners. This is useful in allowing the opportunity for confirmation together with retinal photography and direct discussion with ophthalmologists.

Efficient screening and appropriate and timely referral is very important in order to save eyes from blindness as treatment is most effective if the retinopathy is detected and treated before it has caused symptoms.

5 Management of diabetic retinopathy

Management of diabetic retinopathy should be considered under two headings.

1 The management of the diabetes and associated risk factors with a view to prevention of retinopathy or prevention of progression if already present.

2 The treatment of the eye with sight threatening retinopathy.

Prevention of development and/or progression of retinopathy

Glycaemic control

There is now no doubt that as the glycaemic control of diabetes improves, there is less likelihood of retinopathy (and other microvascular complications) occurring or, if present already, progressing. This has been clearly shown in Type 1 diabetes (IDDM) by the Diabetes Control and Complications Trial (DCCT) and is generally accepted to also be the case in Type 2 diabetes (NIDDM). The DCCT showed a 76% reduction in onset of retinopathy and a 54% reduction in progression of pre-existing retinopathy in patients with normal or near normal glycaemic control. The beneficial effects correlated with HbA1c levels—any improvement of control being found to be beneficial but greatest at the lowest levels. There needs to be caution however. The maintenance of near normal HbA1c levels may lead to significant effects on quality of life from severe hypoglycaemia and hypoglycaemic unawareness. Also, in patients with retinopathy and chronic poor control, care needs to be exercised in improving control because sudden improvements may worsen the retinopathy and changes should therefore be made gently. It should also be remembered that in order to achieve and maintain near normal glycaemic control, considerable resources in time and effort are required by multidisciplinary professional teams and patients themselves—a situation that is not readily achieved or found in normal practice outside the research arena. Suffice it to say however, that the better the control that can be achieved, without compromising general quality of life, the less likely there are to be problems with diabetic retinopathy. Such a programme should be discussed with patients at risk.

Requirements
- Stability of diet and lifestyle
- Intensive insulin regimes in IDDM
- Regular blood glucose monitoring
- Frequent review and discussion
- Open access for help and encouragement
- Annual review screening

Other risk factors and considerations

Hypertension

It is essential to control hypertension to reduce risk of development and progression of retinopathy. This applies also to nephropathy. Blood pressure should be controlled to a normal level of < 140/85. Angiotensin-converting enzyme (ACE) inhibitors are probably the treatment of choice as there is gathering evidence that they may be effective in reducing retinopathy progression even in normotensive people. Caution may be required in NIDDM with generalized vascular disease, with careful monitoring of renal function, because there may be concomitant renal artery stenosis. Combination treatments with ACE inhibitors would include, diuretics, calcium antagonists, beta-blockers or alpha-blockers. The important aim is to maintain normotension.

Pregnancy

Microvascular disease can accelerate in pregnancy and therefore women with diabetes should have their eyes and blood pressure screened every 6 weeks throughout pregnancy.

Smoking

Although there is conflicting evidence regarding smoking as a risk factor for retinopathy in particular, there is incontrovertible evidence regarding its role in vascular disease generally and patients should be strongly advised and encouraged to stop.

Alcohol
Alcohol, provided it is consumed in reasonable amounts and does not cause poor glycaemic control, may have a beneficial effect.

Lipids
Cholesterol and triglyceride levels should be checked and, if abnormal, controlled with lipid lowering agents. This is important not necessarily because of a specific relationship to retinopathy but to reduce the risks of further retinal vascular occlusive events to which people with diabetes are susceptible.

ACE inhibitors
There is gathering evidence that ACE inhibitors reduce the progression of retinopathy even in the absence of microalbuminuria or hypertension.

Aspirin
There is no conclusive evidence that aspirin has a protective effect on retinopathy progression.

Recommended action for anyone with any diabetic retinopathy
- Attain and maintain good metabolic control (HbA1c 7.5% or less)
- Start on ACE inhibitor regardless of any BP elevation
- Control hypertension
- Treat abnormal blood lipid profiles
- Rescreen or refer to ophthalmology as indicated

Treatment of the eye with potentially sight threatening retinopathy

Laser photocoagulation

Retinal laser photocoagulation is currently the mainstay of treatment.

Laser light is usually given through a contact lens and slit lamp. Topical anaesthesia is used and it is an outpatient procedure (Fig. 5.1).

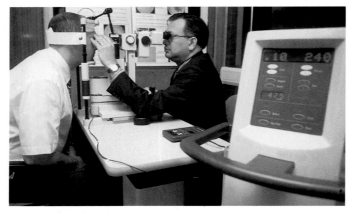

Figure 5.1 Laser treatment.

The aim of laser treatment is to partially destroy ischaemic retina and seal areas of vascular leakage.

The two main indications are proliferative retinopathy and exudative maculopathy or exudates within the temporal vascular arcade. The type of treatment required is quite different.

Proliferative retinopathy

New vessels of proliferative retinopathy are produced in response to an ischaemic retina. Laser treatment is therefore applied, not at the new vessels themselves but at the peripheral retina (Fig. 5.2). Extensive 'Pan-retinal photocoagulation' (PRP) treatment is required with several thousand burns. Further treatments may be required but the new vessels usually regress satisfactorily in 4–6 weeks.

Exudative retinopathy and maculopathy

Exudates represent vascular leakage. Focal laser burns are applied to the area(s) of leakage in the centre of the circinate exudate(s). The exudates should clear within a few months after successful treatment. Laser treatment can also be helpful in some types of macular oedema provided that areas of vascular leakage can be identified by fluorescein angiography. In this situation, laser treatment may be applied in a grid pattern.

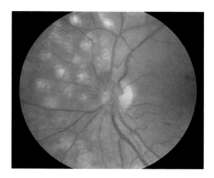

Figure 5.2 Laser treatment scars and proliferative retinopathy (NVD).

Pan-retinal photocoagulation treatment is a destructive process and should be carefully explained to patients who should be given an explanatory leaflet. It should be explained that, although the treatment may cause some loss of the peripheral visual field and colour sensitivity, it is necessary to prevent the inevitable blindness that would occur if left untreated. Very extensive treatment may result in sufficient loss of the visual fields to disallow driving and the Driver and Vehicle Licensing Agency now has strict criteria in this respect.

Vitreoretinal surgery in proliferative retinopathy

Laser treatment is not always completely effective, particularly in advanced disease, and in the presence of persistent vitreous haemorrhage it may not be possible to view the retina adequately. Successful vitreoretinal surgery can now save eyes that would previously inevitably have gone blind. Vitrectomy and intraocular 'endolaser' can salvage such a situation, and any fibrous bands, that would otherwise threaten retinal detachment, can be cut.

There is unfortunately no successful treatment for advanced maculopathy.

Prevention of sight threatening retinopathy is the best solution, and physicians can do much to help, but laser treatment and, if necessary, vitreoretinal surgery, can now save the sight of many people who would, in the past, have inevitably gone blind. Success is dependent upon efficient screening, good diabetes management and adequate eye treatment at an early stage.

6 Management of visual loss

Visual loss cannot always be prevented and people with diabetes are not immune to visual loss from causes other than diabetic retinopathy. However, much can be done to improve the quality of life for people with lost vision and the diabetes care service should not abandon them because the eye disease is no longer treatable. It is important that people with visual impairment from diabetic eye disease continue to be seen for regular review by ophthalmologists.

General considerations

Registration

It is helpful to people with visual loss to be registered, either 'partially sighted' or 'blind' as this will entitle them to benefits. Referral to an ophthalmologist is necessary for registration and they will complete a BD8 form.

Partial sightedness may either be likely to remain stable or be expected to progress to blindness and different benefits may be available depending upon the category. Partial sightedness means sight impairment to an extent where some retraining or rehabilitation may be necessary for employment.

Blindness does not mean that people can see nothing at all, but that vision is sufficiently impaired for the patient to be unable to perform any work for which eyesight is essential. Visual impairment may also affect the ability to drive and to perform essential tasks for daily living.

Criteria for driving:
Minimum legal requirement: ability to read a car number plate with 3.5 inch (8.9 cm) high figures at a distance of 75 feet (22.9 m). This is unlikely to be the case if Snellen chart vision (corrected) is worse than 6/12. Extensive laser treatment may reduce the visual fields and the Driver and Vehicle Licensing Agency may require an examination and report.

Criteria* for registration
Partial sightedness: visual acuity 6/60 or worse in both eyes.
Blindness: visual acuity 3/60 or worse in the better eye.

* Registration can occur with better acuity if there is restriction of the visual fields

When the registration form has been completed it is sent to the Social Services Department and social workers should be available to provide support, practical help and information about local services. A rehabilitation worker will carry out a functional assessment and discuss issues such as employment, finance, mobility, low visual aids, the possibility of learning Braille, etc.

Various allowances and benefits may be available and include:
• unemployment benefit
• statutory sick pay
• incapacity benefit
• income support
• disability premium
• disability living allowance
• mobility allowance
• attendance allowance
• invalidity care allowance
• disabled car and rail cards
  Details are available from: The RNIB Benefit Rights and Information team, RNIB, 224, Great Portland St., London W1N 6AA

Support and counselling services

People with recent or developing visual impairment will require help and support and may wish to express many emotions to the diabetes care team. The team should be prepared for this and should be honest and not give false hopes. They may be able to offer counselling themselves or refer locally. Hospitals often have a nurse counsellor in the eye department. Diabetes care teams should, in any case, always have available information, and names and addresses of local and national people and organizations that can. The BDA publishes a useful booklet.

Counselling
- British Association for Counselling
  1 Regent Place
  Rugby
  Warwickshire
  CV21 2PJ
  01788 578328
- National Diabetes Retinopathy Network (NDRN)
  7 Shore Close
  Hampton
  Middlesex
  PW12 3XS
  0181 9415821
- Relate (previously the National Marriage Guidance Council)
  Herbert Gray College
  Little Church St
  Rugby
  CV21 3AP
  01788 573241

Clearly it is a shattering blow for people to lose vision, but independence and good quality of life can be obtained with the help and support of the many dedicated agencies that are available.

General information
- British Diabetic Association
  10 Queen Anne St
  London
  W1M 0BD
  0171 3231531
- Royal National Institute for the Blind (RNIB)
  224 Great Portland St
  London
  W1N 6AA
  0171 3881266
- RNIB Scotland
  10 Magdala Crescent
  Edinburgh
  E12 5BE
  0131 3131498
- Partially Sighted Society
  Queens Road
  Doncaster
  DN1 2NX

- Guide Dogs for the Blind Association
  Hill fields
  Burfield Common
  Reading
  RG7 3YG
- Action for Blind People
  14–16 Verney Road
  London
  SE16 3DZ
  0171 7328771

Other services

These include:
- Holidays, recreation and rehabilitation advice from the RNIB.
- Talking books (cassettes) from local libraries, RNIB cassette library, Royal National Library for the Blind.
- Talking newspapers from the Talking Newspaper Association of the UK.
- Radio programmes such as BBC Radio 4's *In Touch.*
- Large print, audio and Braille guides from In Touch publishing.

Low visual aids (Fig. 6.1)

A variety of low visual aids are available to help people with visual impairment and range from improved lighting and a simple magnifying glass or magnifying glasses attached to spectacles, through to special computers and closed circuit television. Many simple aids can be bought from optometrists or photographic shops. A low visual aid service will usually be available at the local eye hospital. Various home aids and appliances are also available.

Details can be obtained from the Royal National Institute for the Blind.

Management of the diabetes with associated visual loss

Visual impairment may cause significant difficulties with self-management of diabetes, particularly insulin injections and

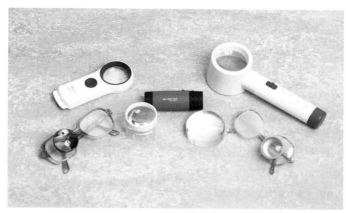

Figure 6.1 Examples of some low visual aids.

blood glucose monitoring. Independence can be maintained by the use of suitable equipment.

Insulin injections

Click count and preset glass insulin syringes are still obtainable but have largely been superseded by the ready availability of insulin pen-injectors (Fig. 6.2). These are now the most convenient way for visually impaired people to manage their insulin. Advice can usually be obtained from specialist diabetes centres and individual patients instructed and advised on the most suitable pen device for them. Alternatively there are insulin vial guides, magnifiers and needle guides available for use with standard plastic syringes and some people may manage satisfactorily with these.

Tablet medication

'Pillminders' are available from the RNIB and some pharmacies (Fig. 6.3). These can be filled periodically by a sighted person and then left for the visually handicapped to safely self-administer their tablets.

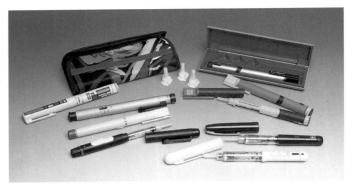

Figure 6.2 A selection of insulin injector pens.

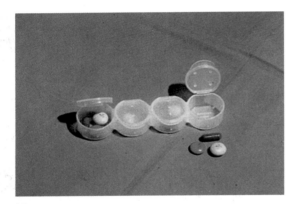

(a)

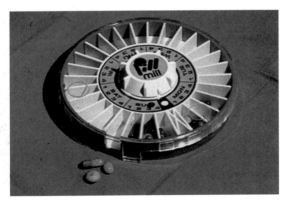

(b)

Figure 6.3 Pill-organizers for visually handicapped people.

Blood glucose monitoring

Many people with partial sight will be able to continue to use ordinary blood glucose meters, perhaps with enhanced lighting and a magnifier. Newer meters have clear digital displays, do not require accurate placing of the blood on the test strip or careful wiping, and are easy to operate. Many will have memories that record and store results for use in future discussion with a diabetes care professional.

There are also meters specially designed for people with visual loss (Fig. 6.4). Some meters such as the Talking Hypocount (Hypoguard) gives a visual display and 'speaks' the result. Others, like the One Touch (Lifescan), can be attached to an accessory module containing a computerized voicebox and this meter also contains a memory to store results for future discussion.

Summary

- People with visual impairment and diabetes can continue to lead a good quality independent life.
- Diabetes care professionals can do much to help and support them and encourage them to utilize the many organizations

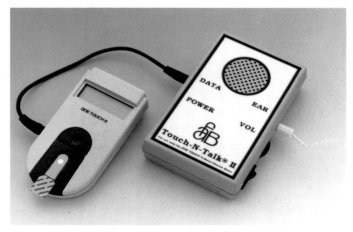

Figure 6.4 A 'talking' blood glucose meter.

and resources available. They should have available the relevant names, addresses and telephone numbers.

- Diabetes care teams should continue to encourage good metabolic control and screening and treatment for other complications and associated disorders.
- People with visual loss from diabetic eye disease should continue to attend specialist ophthalmologists for review.

7 Other commonly seen retinal abnormalities

All practitioners involved in regular ophthalmoscopy and retinal screening are likely to come across a number of retinal conditions that are not directly related to diabetes or diabetic retinopathy. This chapter gives examples of some of these retinal abnormalities.

Macular abnormalities

Drusen (Fig. 7.1)

Drusen or colloid bodies are seen as yellow spots scattered around the macular area. They do not affect vision unless there is also macular degeneration with which there is an association. They may be confused with exudates. They do not require treatment.

Age-related macular degeneration (Fig. 7.2)

Patchy pigmentation is seen at the macula. It is age related and a common form of gradual visual loss in the elderly. There may be associated drusen. There is no effective treatment.

Disciform macular degeneration (Fig. 7.3)

This is caused by scarring from macular haemorrhage and appears as a white scar at the macula. It causes loss of central vision. No treatment is possible by this stage, but if caught early, before scarring develops, laser treatment may be beneficial.

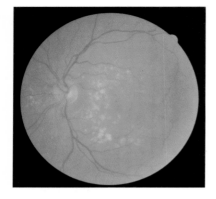

Figure 7.1 Drusen.

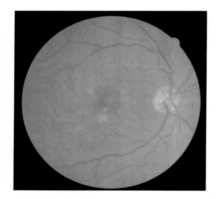

Figure 7.2 Age-related macular degeneration.

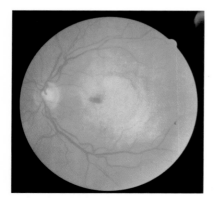

Figure 7.3 Disciform macular degeneration.

Disc abnormalities

Myopic crescent (Fig. 7.4)

In myopia there will be seen a white crescent around the disc and the choroidal vessels are easily visible as if the retina were transparent. There may be associated choroidoretinal degeneration.

Medullated nerve fibres (Fig. 7.5)

This is a harmless congenital abnormality in which a bright white feathery patch is seen due to an extension of the myelin sheaths of the optic nerve fibres beyond the disc. These are usually

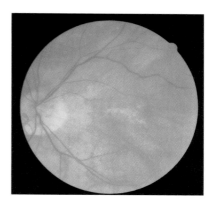

Figure 7.4 Myopic crescent.

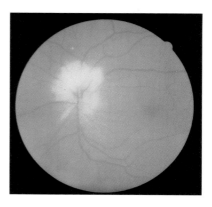

Figure 7.5 Medullated nerve fibres.

seen adjacent to the disc although may occur elsewhere in the retina.

Persistent hyaloid artery

Persistence or a remnant of the hyaloid artery is a not uncommon abnormality which may be confused with neovascularization. A persistent blood vessel or strand of glial tissue may be seen extending from the disc into the vitreous. It is not usually clinically significant.

Coloboma of the retina (Fig. 7.6)

Coloboma is a developmental abnormality and occurs to varying degrees. It may be seen adjacent to the disc. It is seen as a white patch where the sclera is visible through an absent area of retina and choroid.

Papilloedema (Fig. 7.7)

Papilloedema refers to swelling of the disc due to oedema within the optic nerve head. The disc appears swollen and the edges blurred. There may be associated haemorrhages around a hyperaemic disc and venous engorgement. In chronic papilloedema the disc becomes pale. Common causes include raised intracranial pressure and malignant hypertension.

Papillitis (optic neuritis) due to multiple sclerosis or ischaemia

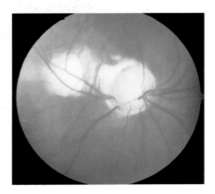

Figure 7.6 Coloboma.

leads to an identical appearance but can be distinguished because there will be a reduction in visual acuity.

It is always pathological and requires investigation.

Optic atrophy

In optic atrophy the disc is abnormally pale and sharply defined. There will be a reduction in visual acuity. It requires a specialist opinion and investigation. This man has an optic nerve glioma (Fig. 7.8).

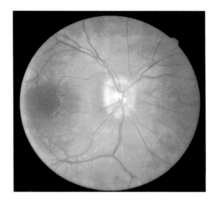

Figure 7.7 Papilloedema.

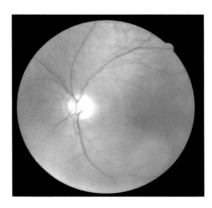

Figure 7.8 Optic atrophy.

Vascular abnormalities

Severe Hypertension (Fig. 7.9)

Flame shaped haemorrhages and cotton wool spots are seen. Hard exudates may also be present around the fovea and seen as a 'macular star'. The term malignant hypertension is used if papilloedema is also present.

Retinal vein occlusions

Central retinal vein occlusion causes sudden loss of vision. Gross dilatation and tortuosity of all retinal veins will be seen with haemorrhages spreading out from and partially obscuring a swollen oedematous disc (Fig. 7.10).

Retinal vein occlusions are seen in association with diabetes, hypertension and hyperviscosity states.

Branch retinal vein occlusions will produce similar, though less dramatic, appearances and confined only to the quadrant of the occluded vein. Haemorrhages, and later exudates, are seen distal to the branch vein occlusion (Figs 7.11 & 7.12).

Retinal artery occlusions

Central retinal artery occlusion produces sudden loss of vision. The retina appears pale due to oedema and the arteries barely visible due to marked narrowing. The macula appears red in

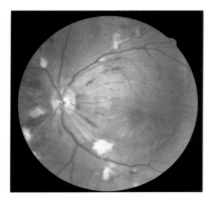

Figure 7.9 Severe hypertensive retinopathy.

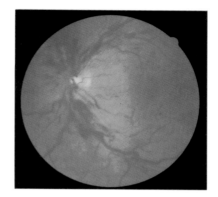

Figure 7.10 Central retinal vein thrombosis.

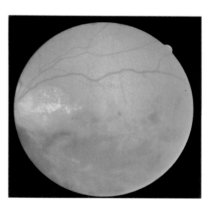

Figure 7.11 Branch retinal vein occlusion (new).

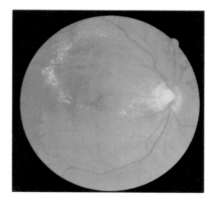

Figure 7.12 Branch retinal vein occlusion (old).

contrast (cherry red spot). At a later stage optic atrophy occurs and the retina appears rather 'empty' of arteries (Fig. 7.13a).

Branch retinal artery occlusions produce the same changes but confined to the area supplied by the occluded branch artery.

'Ghost' empty arteries may be seen in the retina as a sign of past occlusions in people with arteriosclerosis (Fig. 7.13b).

Miscellaneous retinal abnormalities

Congenital tortuosity of the retinal vessels (Fig. 7.14)

The blood vessels are seen to be generally very tortuous in an otherwise fit person. This is a normal variant and not of clinical significance.

Chorioretinitis (Fig. 7.15)

Patches of old chorioretinitis are a common finding and do not require referral or treatment. A patchy area of white scarring with variable degrees of associated pigmentation is seen.

Benign naevus (Fig. 7.16)

Appears as a bluish-grey flat lesion.

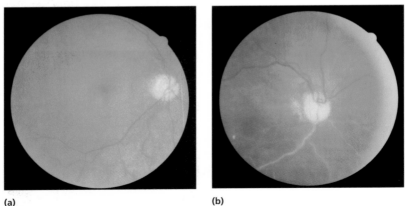

(a) (b)

Figure 7.13 (a) Central retinal artery occlusion. (b) Retinal arterial insufficiency.

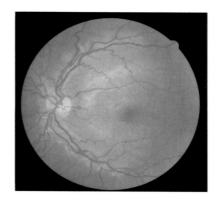

Figure 7.14 Congenital tortuosity of the retinal blood vessels.

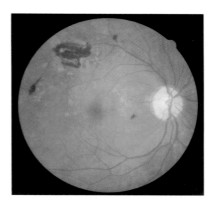

Figure 7.15 Chorioretinitis.

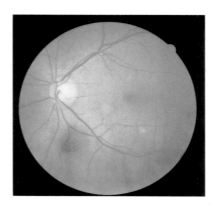

Figure 7.16 Benign naevus.

Malignant melanoma (Fig. 7.17)

Malignant melanoma appears as a raised pigmented area. It is usually seen at the posterior pole of the fundus and there may be an associated retinal detachment.

Retinitis pigmentosa (Fig. 7.18)

This is a hereditary degenerative condition of the retina. The retina has a similar appearance to 'bone histology'.

Retinal pigment epithelial atrophy (Fig. 7.19)

Note the area of depigmentation of the retina, the choroidal

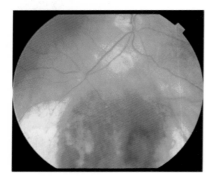

Figure 7.17 Malignant melanoma.

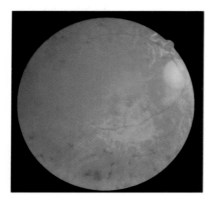

Figure 7.18 Retinitis pigmentosa.

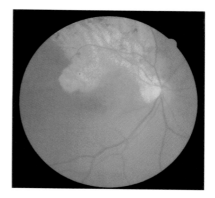

Figure 7.19 Retinal pigment epithelial atrophy.

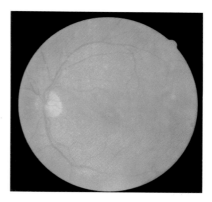

Figure 7.20 Hyaline (asteroid) hyalosis.

vessels are clearly visible beneath this pale atrophic area. No action is required.

Hyaline (asteroid) hyalosis (Fig. 7.20)

Multiple floaters are seen in the vitreous, like a snowstorm in a Christmas novelty. This is not of serious significance but may be noticed by the patient. This can be distinguished from drusen and exudates by being clearly in the vitreous and not on the retina.

Index